TANTRA YOGA
FOR BEGINNERS

TANTRA YOGA
FOR BEGINNERS

Prof. Ravindra Kumar PhD
(SWAMI ATMANANDA)

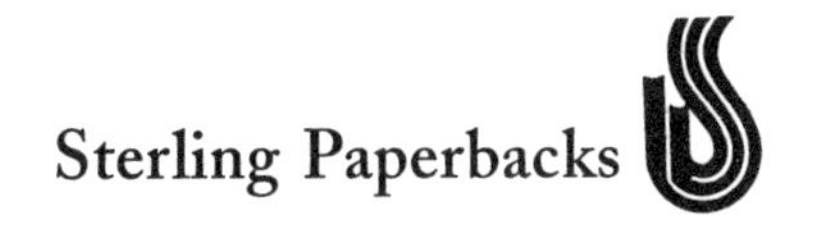

STERLING PAPERBACKS
An imprint of
Sterling Publishers (P) Ltd.
A-59, Okhla Industrial Area, Phase-II,
New Delhi-110020.
Tel: 26387070, 26386209; Fax: 91-11-26383788
E-mail: mail@sterlingpublishers.com
www.sterlingpublishers.com

Originally published under:
All You Wanted To Know About *Tantra Yoga*

Tantra Yoga for Beginners

ISBN 978 81 207 5230 6

Printed in India

Printed and Published by Sterling Publishers Pvt. Ltd.,
New Delhi-110 020.

Contents

Preface

The materialistic or scientific view of time is that objects and events were generated through an origin, way back in time immemorial and that this origin is untraceable. Tantra reverses this viewpoint and believes that objects and events are being produced continuously in the present in the same manner as a flame is projected by the trail-vent of a rocket. The origin is implicit in the projection mechanism and the projection mechanism used by Tantra is sex. Spirituality becomes traceable through this reversal of genesis. This reversal is called *Paravriti* in Sanskrit.

Briefly, the underlying principle of Tantra is to raise one's enjoyment to the highest degree and then use it as a rocket-fuel for spiritual advancement, which eventually leads to enlightenment. The male principle of universal creation is the seed of Being, called Shiva, and the female principle, who is the creative partner, is the goddess Shakti. Shakti spreads out in space, time and the universe before each living being and therefore is nearer for worship than the male principle. She is worshipped in many guises and under many names. Most importantly, she is revered in the form of the female generative organ of the world, that is, the vulva. Tantra recognises the sex-drive and copulation is seen as the symbol of bliss and divine worship. Performed with proper rituals and mantras, it is supposed to be the most powerful tool for achieving enlightenment.

This book provides briefly but sufficiently the necessary knowledge for achieving the goal of enlightenment. A practical formula is presented, which, when followed rigorously, can lead one to success. Important associative wings of Tantra are yoga, meditation and the chanting of mantras. The Academy of Kundalini Yoga and Quantum Soul provides full guidance on them. One is taught about energies in the human body, which most people usually dissipate in their pointless exertions and recreations. The crux of the matter is to arouse passion and then sublimate it, opening thereby the gates of higher consciousness.

The Academy offers theory and methods of practice in all branches of yoga, meditation, and other occult sciences. The emphasis is on achieving yoga (union) of the soul with the Supersoul, which can be done through any of the yogas - Karma, Jnana, Bhakti, Hatha, Kundalini, Tantra and others. These help us to achieve good health, and a disease-free body is, of course, an automatic by-product of this.

Swami Atmananda (Ravindra Kumar PhD)
Founder President, Academy of Kundalini Yoga and Quantum Soul.
58-61 Vashisht Park, Pankha Road
New Delhi-110046
Tel: 504 7091, 504 7089
E-mail: ravijytte@now-india.net.in
And,
Sofus Francks Vaenge 6,6
DK 2000, Frederiksberg, Denmark
Tel: (45) 36 16 92 50
Email: JytteRavi.Kumar@mail.tele.dk

Introduction

In India, from the Vedic times, a variety of methods have been designed for attaining enlightenment. Tantra is claimed to be the fastest of them all. It begins with the recognition of the sex drive and aims at transcending it. In fact, all methods lay stress on eradication of sex from within the individual, which then opens the way for God to come in. Thus transcendence of sex is an essential step before the attainment of enlightenment. Just as "iron cuts iron" and "a thorn removes a thorn" in the same manner it is "sex that transcends sex". And with this goal in mind, it can be said that all other methods are comparable to the slow speed of a bullock cart, while Tantra is comparable to a fast-moving helicopter. Although it is risky like the helicopter, it can work safely if proper precautions are taken and if performed under guidance. From ancient times, specially endowed female initiators have been the partners in advanced sexual rituals. The temples of Khajuraho in Central India have been there for centuries and depict the technique of transcending sex. Tantric pictures engraved on the temple walls, stimulate a special kind of mental activity, which invokes psychosomatic forces. These forces can transform a person completely, providing him or her with a new basis for life. Even constant staring at these pictures does not arouse any feeling of vulgar sex. Rather sexual feelings are wiped out from the mind, giving way to subtler religious thoughts.

Tantrics arouse all the energies discovered in the body, heart and mind, and combine them into a vehicle, which leads to enlightenment. They use every possible means, adapting every possible emotional stimulus and act to their purpose.

One assumes that things which one actually does repeatedly, and which have associated with them a powerful sensuous and emotive charge, transforms one far more effectively than anything else. Furthermore, the change is radical only when one combines various kinds of doings. This kind of change is fundamental and total.

The four main components of Tantra are yoga, offerings, meditation and copulation. A successful combination of them, for a specific period of time, changes a person forever. It introduces one to a world which can only be accessed by following the maps drawn by the tantric. Someone who has not visited it can have no idea of what it is like. One cannot examine it from the outside. By following the tantric principles, one can be in a position to experience truth about oneself and one's world, just as one can directly see and appreciate the Taj Mahal. A complete transformation of personality is required to attain this position, where one can experience the truth. As said earlier, this requires every kind of effort - physical, mental, sexual and moral. Tantra does not advocate abstinence from all enjoyment, mortification of one's flesh and fear of God's punishment. On the contrary, it advocates that joy be raised to the highest pinnacle and then used as fuel for spiritual advancement. This results in knowledge of truth about the origin of things and humans. This is called enlightenment.

Tantric Model of Genesis

The tantric model confronts the question of time directly. By studying the nature of time, one can understand the process of genesis, and the origin of the cosmos. Once this concept is understood, one can traverse back the ladder of genesis and reach the origin.

According to the materialistic or scientific view of time, one looks backward in time, as if looking at the objects out of the rear window of a moving motor car. We know people who have died, people who are with us at present, and some who existed long ago in history, and then we know some objects, like the earth, which have always existed. According to astronomy, in this kind of notion of time, the world might have had an infinitely remote beginning, which is the central vanishing point of our view of things. Cause and effect gradually connected all objects to each other. However, we might not have really experienced what all these objects represent. Our perception of things is shaped by scientific knowledge. We do not have the direct experience of what the past was or what the lives of the people in the past were like. Furthermore, we ourselves are becoming objects under the law of cause and effect. For example, after death, in the imagination of others, one would appear in the same way as when alive. The whole picture appears like a personal mental fiction, supported by fragments that can be called facts. In fact, it is only the contents of our own memory, which we really know.

Tantra reverses the common sense view of objects and events in the past, emanating from the origin as a landscape in which an individual moves with his "present frame." Tantra thinks of the past as a trail of things and events being projected from the mouth of the present, as if a rocket is projecting the flames from its tail-vent. Such a reversal of genesis is termed *Paravriti* in Sanskrit, which means "turning back up." So here, time and things did not "begin" at some imaginary point or origin, but they are being projected by each of us. The "present frame" of every individual is itself the tail-vent of the rocket which is projecting his or her world of experience and knowledge. In the common sense method, it may never be possible to find the origin (the first cause of all things), while in Tantra, the origin lies in the projection-mechanism itself. In other words, the psychophysical organism itself contains the origin. The projected things and events is the reality, containing experience and memory and appearing solid, as if it had a beginning far back in time. Several icons, called *yantra*, are physical images carrying a charge of symbolism. They focus the thoughts of the tantric on the phases of genesis in time, as and when he worships them. The icons use either sexual symbolisms or human shaped imagery, which convey intuitions of inner states with which the male or female tantric can identify himself or herself. All symbols used in icons or *yantras* are feminine and active at once. Most of the images are varying representations of the *yoni* (vulva), the female organ that generates world and time. They are so dense and real that they convey very exciting emotional realities which seem to be more real than the objects of everyday experience. Some *yantras* are quite complex, Shri yantra being the greatest of them.

Yantra diagrams of various kinds represent the backward look into the rocket spewing out time and space. Meditation on such a *yantra* drives the mind to take that backward look, reversing the act of genesis, and staring straight into the "continuing act of creation." The whole of Tantra revolves around this process. This possibility is kept continuously in mind through an attitude of devotion or reverence to the symbolic images.

The "practical mechanism" used by Tantra to represent the act of projection is "sex." "Sexual activity" is infused with "totally transcendent love" and it expresses the "act of continuous creation." The *yoni* (vulva) of the female principle results from a continuous infusion of the seed of the male in sexual delight.

The *yoni*, in turn, gives birth to the existent world, continuously. The rocket is thus represented by the *yoni* spewing the world out. However, the existence of the *yoni* and the world comes from the seed, which gives the possibility of existence of the whole system. This fact is beyond perception, although it is implicit in the system.

The whole system, including the *yoni*, is originated by the "seed", represented by a point having no dimensions at the centre of the *yantra*. The fundamental originating movement of the seed is the creation of the *yoni*, represented by a downward pointing triangle. The point representing the seed is white, while the triangle representing the *yoni* is red. This original couple of white and red generates a series of interwoven triangles, four upward-pointing males and four downward-pointing females. Many lesser triangles are in turn produced by the interpenetration of major triangles. Lesser triangles represent sub-divisions of original creative energies into specified forces. Rings and outer circles of the lotus petals represent the reality of the world as it unfolds. The creative process works beyond the flow of time, and has all its different phases working simultaneously.

The two creative functions of Brahma, the Absolute Being or the Supreme Truth, are *Mahakala* and *Mahakali*. *Mahakala* is the male personification of time and *Mahakali*, the female one. Everything that exists in the universe is a production of these two. All the objects, however dense they may be, such as humans, rocks and planets are a result of an encounter between fields of energy. They appear to be outside us, but they are in fact so intimately interwoven with human ideas of them that they are inseparable. All objects result from the collision and collusion of forces, which are the sub-functions of time.

Importance of Women in Tantra

Tantra has a male aspect of Brahma, which is hidden and not so easily approachable, and a female aspect, which manifests itself in various forms and is approachable. The female Goddess of time generates us as time-bound entities. Accordingly, we all are closer to the "female aspect of creation." It is therefore easier to meditate on the female to reach the intuitive truth. So, either one worships a female icon, such as a downward-pointing triangle, resembling the female genitals, a lotus-flower and a lingam in an egg-like shape, or, one adores an image of the Goddess representing her as a beautiful girl. The girl in the image dances with crazy love, sometimes lowering her hair to represent the spreading out of the worlds and sometimes binding her hair to represent the end of the worlds. In the 1980s, my *kundalini* got activated and I visualised one such image of a dancing girl in my dreams. However, the image for worship can be in metal, wood, stone or any other thing. Although every woman appears to be clothed in the Goddess, it is the Goddess in the woman who attracts the tantric's attention, and not the woman who personifies the Goddess. In every woman and in every artistic icon one sees the "charm of the inner image," which is intensified in the mind of the tantric. The woman in flesh or other material forms does not imprison one. The role women play in Tantra is very important, since they are carriers of female energy, which is crucial for the tantric. As Philip Rawson says, "Man and woman must continually fulfil and complete each other. Only after a long experience of mutual exchange can either carry out complete tantric rituals alone." In rituals the man and the woman have to cooperate with and complement each other. Every act of human love is a reflection of cosmic love, and its closeness to the divine primal act depends on how completely it is carried out.

The Goddess is responsible for our creation as well as for our destruction. Exterminating the population through epidemics like cholera and AIDS, or through disasters like that which befell the Titanic, or through famine and war, is the destructive side of the same Mother. As an image this is shown as the terrible Goddess Kali, with a black face, a lolling tongue and blood dribbling from her mouth. Many rituals are performed on cremation grounds (real or symbolic) in the red light of funeral pyres, with crows and jackals crunching and scattering the bones, to understand the dissolution of everything that one possesses. Some such rituals include sex too. Her benevolent nature is depicted through the image of Goddess Durga. To become a complete tantric, one has to understand both aspects of the Goddess properly.

The Whole and Creation

The philosophical propositions of the creative process can be easily understood in human and erotic symbolism in the points given below:

(1) Ultimate reality is originally the all-embracing whole, complete in itself with male and female aspects in such a perfect balance that there is no awareness of it. Only "bliss" and "oneness" exists. This is the state of "I"-ness.

(2) Reality divides the sexual pair into the 'male principle being' called Shiva and the 'female principle being' called Shakti. Shiva, as the first stage of creation, has projected Shakti. Shiva is the first cause and as the principle of self and complete identity is the dominant one. The two are so deeply joined that they are unaware of their differences and are

beyond time. The division takes place both within the man and the world. Shakti has her eyes closed in total bliss, since she is not yet awoken to the state of separateness.

(3) The sexual pair becomes aware of their distinction. Shakti's eyes have opened; nevertheless, the two are still united with each other. Shakti is now in the state of separation, which has been realised for the first time. Although the separation was planned and initiated by Shiva, it is Shakti (who was projected specifically for this purpose) who has worked it out. The two face each other, still in embrace, but aware of their separateness.

(4) The couple moves out of union into distinct parts. However, their sexual attraction to each other reminds them of their oneness. They remember that they belong to each other, and that the self and the world are complementary parts of each other. Shakti now begins to function independently.

(5) Shakti operates as the beautiful female dancer, the dance weaving the fabric of the

world. The dance is neither illusory nor real. The fascinated self erroneously believes the different movements and gestures of the dancing Shakti to be different things. Because of the bewildering activity of Shakti, the self begins to think that it is not one but many males and females. Our mind and body present the psychosomatic mechanism to the self in such a way that each of our separated selves appears to be isolated and imprisoned. Such is a bewildering array of infinite and separate facts of which the universe appears to be composed, and that is how we grasp it. This is basically the activity of the Goddess, represented by her fertile womb. That womb has generated the whole course of our individual life, including various things which we experience from time to time. If we could know the truth, we would understand that this dance, this womb and these objects are not different from what we are. All our sense organs and faculties of perception are the channels through which Shakti is working towards separation and distinction. This is in fact the holistic view, which is closer to the ideas, which our present-day science is groping with. According to this philosophy, the "wholes" come first and generate their parts - atoms, molecules, elements, limbs and organs. Every cause, therefore, lies in the whole and not in its parts. Tantric enlightenment is then the "understanding" that the holistic picture combined with time represents the ultimate whole.

(6) This is the tantric scheme of genesis. By traversing back the steps therein, one can climb the ladder of evolution and realise the whole truth. The laboratory for the experiment is one's own body with the senses and experiences. It can be said that the whole universe is contained in the human body, which can be realised through intuition alone. On several occasions some "divine beings" have shown to others the whole universe - stars, planets and creatures contained within their body. The most

notable of these divinities has been Lord Krishna, some five thousand years ago.

(7) In the Indian tantric system, the human body is visualised as an inverted tree with its ground in the beyond, and the Supreme Brahma, the truth. As the nourishing juices are carried upwards in the plants through their channels and veins, even so the creative energies are carried in the human body – the root of the human plant being in the skull (at the top), called *sahasrara* or the crown centre. The energy from beyond passes through the *sahasrara* into the body. Having flown through the body's channels, the nourishing energy flows to the outermost tips of the senses, and then into the space around it, in the form of an aura. The system of the veins and channels through which the energy flows is called the subtle body. There are seven levels of separation between Shiva and Shakti, beginning with *sahasrara* out at the top of the head and ending with *mooladhara* at the base of the spine. These levels are called *chakras* situated along the spinal column. This

path is traversed back from *mooladhara* to *sahasrara* by the mechanism called *kundalini.* The *kundalini* lies dormant at the base of the spine in an average individual. Through tantric practices it is awakened and then it passes through the seven *chakras* from *mooladhara* to *sahasrara*. The arrival of *kundalini* at the crown centre is solemnised as the meeting of Shiva and Shakti and the practitioner goes into *samadhi* and experiences "bliss and enlightenment." This is the end of the journey and all the tantric practices. From now onwards one hears the "Cosmic sound" internally, which connects the soul with the supersoul-Brahma. This stage is also called self-realisation.

The basic difference between ordinary Indian traditions and Tantra is that other traditions preach asceticism and repression of all faculties of the mind and body to experience truth, while Tantra works in the opposite way. In Tantra all the faculties - the senses, the emotions and the intellect - are aroused to the highest level so that the stored memories and responses are awakened and converted back into the originating pure energy. Pleasures and sense enjoyments serve as the raw material for transformation, eventually producing enlightenment. With proper direction and precautions or with the guidance of a realised guru, this is the best-known shortest path to self-realisation. Innumerable examples of successful journeys are available in India, Nepal, Tibet and other countries. However, when direction and guidance are missing, one may fall pray to the trap and may be caught in indulgence, resulting in the wastage of creative energy. People desirous of practising Tantra are always given this warning and advice. One can compare the ordinary methods with a slow bullock cart, while Tantra is the fast method of the helicopter, which of course requires precaution and guidance. The choice lies with each individual. Just as no two persons have the same fingerprints, similarly no two practitioners will follow exactly the same method for self-realisation. Jiddu Krishnamurti has talked about it very clearly at great length.

Techniques of Re-Conversion

Although there are several techniques which overlap each other, the central idea is to use sexual intercourse to reverse the process of creation, as described earlier. A man and a woman who are spiritual partners, sharing a common goal of enlightenment, get into the process carefully so that they are converted back into the personifications of Shiva and Shakti, consummating their union eventually. The period of copulation is prolonged as much as possible, with regular practice, so that eventually all intermediate stages are crossed and the two blend into each other, experiencing the condition which existed prior to the separation. There is tremendous pleasure and bliss, taking the couple to beyond genesis. Tantric couples engaged in yogic sex leading to spiritual fulfilment have been pictured in the Buddhist art of Tibet as a symbol of enlightenment.

Techniques that support and encourage tantric sex towards perfection are mainly—yoga, chanting of mantras and offerings to an image, among some others. Let us begin with yoga, which is an important constituent in the process. Although there are various kinds of yogas, it is certain specific postures of Hatha yoga, which are very useful. Yogic exercises have to be coupled with inner work with the subtle body; only then does it go beyond simply improving physical health. Body actions in yogic exercises are nearly the same as those in sexual intercourse. There are yogic postures which provide pressure, contractions, expansions, pulls and twists to certain muscles which are strengthened in order to perform better and prolonged sex, and they hold ejaculation for a considerable period of time. Physical sensations are enhanced and they induce blissful insight. There are trained and experienced persons who teach the tricks of the game to their partners, under the guidance of a teacher or otherwise. Generally, there are trained women teachers who initiate the males into the process. There are innumerable examples of well-known male saints who were initiated through sexual intercourse by "power-holding women."

Later religions in India are all male-oriented, but in ancient times female-power was more prominent. There used to be a lineage of power-holding women, whose favour the male practitioners had to win, in order to earn an initiation. Writers of present themes in Tantra have consistently tried to play down the role of such women. The male practitioner would have sexual relations with women whose charms would arouse them and this would lead to tantric sex and enlightenment. There used to be family prostitutes, temple dancers and singers, who were not experts in sexual intercourse and tantric rituals. But they attracted the male practitioners sexually and become prime agents in their spiritual advancement. Such women normally belonged to low castes, and relationships with them brought down male practitioners in the eyes of society. However, men liked it, since they wanted to break all ties with conventional society, in order to get enlightenment. To continue to be respectable men in society was a bondage, which could be an obstacle in the path of spiritual advancement. Accordingly, lovers of spiritual enlightenment would live practically as social exiles as most people in society would not be practitioners of Tantra. Many famous saints, sages, writers and poets belong to this category. Dr. B. Bhattacharya, who has authored many books on Tantra, such as, *Towards a Tantric Goal* (1989) is a present-day tantric. Dr. Bhattacharya describes in detail his sexual relationship with a tantric female, whom he calls LS, in order to conceal her identity. He was initiated by LS through sexual intercourse and he eventually acquired tantric enlightenment. Dr. Bhattacharya, probably in his late 80s or early 90s, was still living in Delhi when this book was being written.

The best time to have tantric sex with a woman is when she is menstruating, since her "red sexual energy" is at its peak then. The intercourse becomes more rewarding if it is carried out in the cremation ground, around the flaming pyres of a corpse. There are two schools of thought about this. One of them says that the "white male seed" should be ejaculated in the *yoni* as a sacrifice; and the orgasms of both the partners prolonged by long yogic practices transforms into ecstasy of the highest order. According to the other school of thought, the orgasms should be restrained and sublimated, and the passions thus created should be directed towards higher centres, opening thereby the gates of higher perception. In either of these ways, the goal can be achieved. In fact, it could be a combination of both, in variations. This is so because one can hold the seed for a long time, and then it can be sublimated. When it becomes impossible to hold the seed after a few successful attempts and ejaculation becomes essential, then it should be ejaculated in the *yoni*, as a sacrifice.

In a ritual called *chakrapuja*, which involves a group of males and females, who may or may not be married, couples indulge in five kinds of pleasures – meat, alcohol, fish, a particular grain and sexual intercourse. Passions and pleasures are aroused to the maximum, and then again, either the orgasms are sublimated, or the semen is collected in one container and then tasted by everyone as the blessed item. There are different ways suggested by different schools of thought, but each one of them appears to be a potential way of achieving the goal. In many old texts the "snake" is used to represent "cosmic and creative sexual energy". The snake represents *kundalini*. The tantric method can be seen as the fastest way of arousing *kundalini* by its followers.

Other methods which aid tantric transformation and make it work faster are offerings to images and chantings of mantras, as mentioned earlier. One chooses an image of one's own liking, which is worthy of worship. For example, it could be a *yantra* or a succession of images, including even a live girl, into whom the Goddess descends as a whole. The image may be made of paper, mud or some permanent material. With dedication and reverence the practitioner identifies self with the image and concentrates upon it. The image is given a bath, touched with coloured powder, garlanded and offered green leaves, flowers, incense, light and food – all that which responds to the senses. All this is done to "welcome the guest" into the house and oneself. It is understood that when the image is worshipped as such, it acquires power and value in course of time. One could say that cosmic energy begins to dwell in there. All this is very meaningful, if understood in the right way.

Next and perhaps one of the most important methods of empowerment is the chanting of a mantra, which is a carefully selected garland of syllables in Sanskrit. A mantra contains the energy of the related deity, in seed form. There are various mantras tested by *yogis* over the years and are available to the practitioners. The practitioner has to understand the meaning of the mantra and learn the correct pronunciations, before chanting it. The mantras are used throughout the ritual in the form of a whisper or in different combinations and contexts, so as to create a "vibrating pattern," which condenses the related energy at the time and place of the ritual. On repeated chanting of the mantra for a considerable period of time, this latent energy precipitates and the apparition of the deity appears in human-consciousness. This is actual manifestation of cosmic energy in the cherished form of the practitioner, which overwhelms him or her with immense happiness and bliss. This can be said to be a happening of the highest order, in which God manifests Himself in human form for the satisfaction of His devotee. This is how I saw Mother Goddess appearing before me and blessing me with her right hand, moving it over my head with a pleasing smile. It happened three times in a period of about two months in the year 1987. However, it is not necessary to undergo all tantric rituals for experiencing the power of a mantra; in other words, proper chanting of mantras alone is powerful enough to reach the goal of enlightenment.

In fact, all kinds of artistic experiences are cultivated in Tantra, for their own sake. All the body's stored up responses - emotional, sensuous and intellectual - which can produce an arousal, are used as fuel to the flame of Tantra. One can mention here the stimulating beauty of erotic temple sculpture and poetry reading and musical performances. According to tantric belief, the great Goddess projects herself into Krishna and Radha in order to give a taste of cosmic ecstasy to positive lovers. The practitioner combines different methods of transformation — offerings to an image, chanting of mantras, yoga and sexual intercourse—in variation. One acquires a "radiant inner condition" when successful in his or her tantric practices.

The Subtle Body

The reversal of the process of genesis works through the inner body, which is subtle. The "subtle body" has knots and veins through which the currents of energy flow in the psychosomatic system of humans. This body does not belong to the outer world of objective facts, but it is experienced inwardly and is more real than the objects of the physical world. One can experience the subtle body by focusing one's attention inwardly. Hindu and Buddhist seekers agree on the existence and functioning of the subtle body. The practitioner concentrates inwardly on the whole — as a *mandala,* with mythical Mount Meru at the centre and other parts of the worlds around it. He/she visualises the revolving planets and heavens in the *mandala*. This can lead his perception of things

Gentle Leader
dog harness - Blitz

to a higher level. A tantric practitioner keeps track of the events of his/her life through the study of occult sciences, such as astrology, numerology, palmistry and astronomy.

One's spinal column is compared with the central axis of Mount Meru, and the whole world is visualised as revolving around oneself. One visualises the whole cosmos and all individuals emanating from one's own sensuous and mental structure, and focuses them upon the lower *chakras* in one's body. There are seven *chakras* or vortices of vital energy, along the spinal column. The *chakras* are shown as lotuses in the diagrams, which are stationed along the central nerve *sushumna* on the spinal column. On both sides of the central nerve there are two other nerves *-pingla* (male, white and related to the sun) and *ida* (female, red and related to the moon) - which entwine around these lotuses and are responsible for circulating the energy. There are seven *chakras*, starting from the root-*chakra* (between the anus and genitals), and travelling upwards to the sacral-*chakra* (near the end of the tail bone), the naval-*chakra* (near the solar plexus), the *anahat-chakra* (near the centre of the chest), the throat-*chakra* (near the throat-pit), and the eyebrow-*chakra* (at the mid-point between the eyebrows), and ending with the crown-*chakra* (near the centre of the head). There is female creative energy called *kundalini,* which lies dormant near the base of the spine, like a fine snake in three-and-a-half coils, closing the opening of *sushumna* with its mouth. With intense tantric practices *kundalini* gets aroused one day, and after passing the six *chakras* arrives at the seventh *chakra* at the crown centre. Awakening *kundalini* is the main purpose of tantric practices. When it awakens, one hears a hissing sound like that of a snake or a sound like the blowing of a conch, which becomes a permanent feature with inner hearing.

Kundalini touches the crown and returns. Great care must be taken that the ascension does not take place through *ida* or *pingla,* which is erroneous. If *kundalini* ascends through *ida,* there is excessive coolness produced in the practitioner; while if it ascends through *pingla,* there is excessive heat produced; both situations are not desirable. The practitioner in such a case has to find some advanced *yogi* to help, or make repeated efforts to undo the ascension and attempt re-ascension through *sushumna*. Dr. B. S. Goel, author of *Third Eye and Kundalini* (1985) and working as a guru in his ashram near Delhi was a victim of wrong ascension for which he suffered for about nine years. With repeated efforts *kundalini* is made to ascend the *sushumna* as often as possible, and then eventually reside there permanently, as a symbol of Shiva and Shakti having united forever. A Hindu tantric recognises the ascension of kundalini with tingling sensuous movements, just like the crawling of a snake or the leaps of a frog. A Buddhist tantric recognises the same by the ascension of an "inner girl" represented by the red Goddess Dakini. The ascension of *kundalini* is neither a Hindu nor a Buddhist event, and the practitioner may experience either or both kinds of symptoms. I personally experienced both which is described in my book, *Kundalini-An Autobiographical Guide to Self/God Realization* (1999).

Enlightenment or Self-Realisation

Arrival of *kundalini* at the crown centre is described as female energy (Shakti) meeting and uniting with its male counterpart (Shiva) sexually. This union results in the flow of nectar, which floods the whole body of the practitioner leading to immense pleasure and bliss, incomparable with anything in the physical world. The nearest "partial approximation" can be the experience associated with orgasm in sexual intercourse. It is at this point that "human sexuality" gets converted into "divine sexuality," which is the aim of tantric practices. The man or the woman who experiences this union becomes "whole" and is identified with the origin or the source of self and world, near the crown centre. The chain of reincarnations is broken and one moves as a happy desireless whole person, called *jeevanmukta* or "liberated while still living." There are many symbols by which this union is recognised in different faiths and traditions, for example, the mystical great bird Simurg of Persia, carrying a pair of divine lovers. Hindus represent it as the half-male-half-female figure of Shiva and Shakti, called *ardhanaareeshwara*. The same thing is represented by a hermaphrodite being in Judaism and Gnosticism, and by an androgynous being in Greek mythology. This is the goal of humanity and all faiths and traditions of the world. Of course, there are a variety of methods to achieve this goal.

The reversal of genesis is affected by the ascent of *kundalini* through the five elemental states of matter - solid (symbolised by earth), liquid (by water), incandescent (by fire), gaseous (by air), and ether (by itself). Each higher state of matter corresponds to more intense inner perception in the practitioner. Just as one passes from childhood to youth to old age, without a clear age of demarcation, even so, the yogi passes from *savikalpa samadhi* to *asampragyata* to *nirvikalpa samadhi*; in fact, one passes from old age to astral existence through the gateway of death in the same manner. Each state fuses into the next without any clear line of separation, since there is none in reality. You cannot say when childhood ends or when boyhood or youth begins, or when youth ends and old age begins; it is just a continuous process. Even so, the *yogi* passes from one stage to another in *samadhi*; without being aware of it, it just goes on happening. Tantric Buddhists represent these stages of transition by a variety of domed mounds called stupas, varying in size from a small metallic object to a huge building.

Corresponding to the seven *chakras*, Hindu Tantra has divided the states of inner development into seven divisions. The location of the *chakras* has already been discussed earlier. The first *chakra* called *mooladhara* represents the solid state having a yellow colour and a square shape and four petals in a lotus. The second *chakra* called *swadhishthan* represents the liquid state having a white colour and a circular shape, and six petals in a lotus. The third *chakra* called *manipura* represents the fiery state having a red incandescent colour and a triangular shape, and eight petals in a lotus. The fourth *chakra* called *anahata* represents the airy state having a green colour and a semi-lunar shape, and twelve petals in a lotus. The fifth *chakra* called *vishuddhi* represents the ethereal state having a gray colour and a wisp-like shape, and sixteen petals in a lotus. The sixth *chakra* called *ajna* is the place beyond ether where the ego is fragmented into a thousand pieces, and where the union of male and female is consummated. *Ajna* has two petals in the white lotus, and its activation opens the gateway to liberation. The seventh *chakra* called *sahasrara* has the radiance of the sum total of all colours and has a thousand petals in the lotus. When the inner state of the practitioner arrives at this level, he/she is already not of the world, although living in the world. He/she is liberated while still living, and his/her body can really drop down anytime unless some interest keeps him/her alive on earth. According to one school of thought, an additional *chakra* is situated just below the heart and is called the “island of jewels”. It is here that the sense of a separate self is generated in the individual during involution, and obliterated during evolution. The downward course of genesis can be called involution and the upward return can be called evolution.

Buddhist Tantra

Buddhist Tantra does not recognise the first *chakra mooladhara* and *kundalini*. However, it identifies the ascending energy of consciousness with sex power, in the form of male semen being borne by the female. It recognises the *chakra* at the naval region as the critical stage of transformation like Hindu Tantra. Corresponding to the dead body in a funeral pyre, this *chakra* immolates the self in the presence of the flaming guardian deities. The next *chakra* at the level of the heart is of utmost importance in Buddhism, where the set is divided in five circles in the five directions – east, west, north, south, and the fifth, which is at the centre. Each circle has in it a peaceful Buddha, in sexual union with his consort "Wisdom", in the state of meditation. Each of the figures represents a particular "mistaken sentimental view" and a "deluding mental function". These are inverted by the grace and wisdom of the female with whom the Buddha is sexually united. In systematic succession, the practitioner should identify himself with each Buddha, thereby opening the mind by the grace of the associated "Wisdom", and eventually reaching the state of full realisation. Buddhist philosophy believes in the abandonment of all objects, lower or higher, dissolving them one by one as one's illusions, finally reaching the spaceless and timeless "void".

The set of five fields - south, east, north, west and centre, each containing a Buddha in sexual union with his consort, and representing a particular human drawback, is to be meditated upon by the practitioner in the above spiral order. For example, the one in the east represents the important emotion "anger", which upon meditation on the image is helped by the deity Vajrapani (one who holds the *vajra* - a steel implement). This negative emotion is eradicated from within the practitioner. In this way one completes the round and transcends one's negative emotions. Next, he comes to the central *sushumna* through which his consciousness-energy rises to the throat centre. It is here that he encounters a similar field of deities holding knowledge, and each corresponding to a Buddha in sexual union with his consort. Once again the practitioner passes through the fields in the same spiral order, transcending one's negative energies and gaining new knowledge. After completing this round at the throat centre, once again the consciousness-energy rises to the highest centre and a similar procedure is followed. At this level the negative energies are of the highest order, possessing violent passion - wrathful as well as sexual. Completion of this round transcends one above all negative passion and opens one to the Supreme Knowledge. Either a golden couple or a blue Buddha sitting in a peaceful sexual embrace with his female Wisdom in pure white depicts this level of transcendence. Sets of *yantras* with varying shapes and colours are also used to represent this whole system.

Use of a mantra is very effective in the process. One continuously chants the mantra *"Om Mani Padme Hum"*, representing the state of completeness — *Om* is the primordial sound connecting the soul to the Supersoul. *Mani* means "jewel". *Padme* means "in the lotus" and *Hum* is the powerful sound that forces the mantra into realisation. "Jewel in the lotus" is the symbolic representation of *"lingam* in the *yoni"*, representing the final tranquil state of oneness, from where everything started in the beginning. This is the final rest and end of Tantra. Each Buddhist tantric holds a *vajra* (two-pronged steel implement), which symbolises the energy of the mantra. Sometimes the tantric uses a bell, such that its rim is constantly rubbed with a stick producing a humming sound that helps in the progression of meditation. This sound is an approximation of the primordial unstruck sound of *Om*. According to the tantric belief the significance of sound lies in the philosophy that every object is related to a particular vibration. The correct chanting of *Om*, over a period of time, can actually generate the basic sound of

Om, and connect the soul with the Absolute. This would be the culmination of all tantric practices, including meditation, devotional activities, sexual yoga and the chanting of mantras. One can actually ride over the current of *Om* and arrive at the centre of God.

Freedom from Lust

It is the most powerful, most natural and perhaps the shortest path to Self/God realisation, if it is understood properly. "The tantric tried to transform sex into spirituality but the preachers of morality, in our country, did not allow the message to reach the masses". Although thinking about Tantra was banned thousands of years ago, its philosophy is immortalised in the monuments of Khajuraho and the temples of Puri and Konark in India. Seeing the images of naked couples in intercourse, on the outer walls of the Khajuraho temple, one does not feel any sense of vulgarity; rather, one is enveloped in the feelings of sacredness and peace. On the faces of the statues one will find the serene and peaceful impression of Buddha and Mahavira. The visionaries who knew spiritual sex intimately created the statues. Just as watching two men fight satisfies and dissipates the instinct of fight deep rooted in a man, meditation on these images of intercourse evaporates mad sexuality from within and one becomes calm and peaceful. Freedom from lust can be achieved through long sessions of concentration on these drawings. After freeing oneself from the sexuality of the outer walls and on entering the temple, one sees the peaceful statue of Lord Shiva instituted inside. This is the secret of Tantra.

If one observes the process of copulation and orgasm closely, one would find that two things are created in those depths - egolessness and timelessness; and these are the characteristics of *samadhi*. In that brief moment of sexual climax, the individual tastes bliss and divinity. To have the same experience again, the person indulges in sex repeatedly and loses a considerable amount of energy and vitality. One later regrets one's indulgence and laments the loss. However, one has touched the subtler level of the sexual experience, which is religious in essence. What one has to understand at this point is that "sexual pleasure" is not the "end" but the "means" to attain the permanent bliss of *samadhi*. Normally, ejaculation accompanies orgasm. If one can know the secret of separating "ejaculation" from "orgasm", one will not lose the energy and vitality on the one hand, and enjoy the "bliss" of the Absolute on the other. This is what happens to the *yogis*. They are in a state of permanent bliss and full of energy. This is where meditation comes into the picture and one is required to know the art of converting sex into meditation.

The act of sexual union gives man a chance to be influenced by the force which is properly human because during the moment of orgasm, the innermost self of the man or woman becomes isolated from the lower forces. At this instant, if a man can be free of desire and of thinking, he will become aware of an inner awakening to his true nature."

When one's consciousness is raised to a purely human level in the sexual act, one can become aware of the nature of the lower forces and can detach oneself from them. Once their domination is over, the person becomes their master and then one can direct them to their proper paths.

From Sexuality to Spirituality

According to Swami Satyananda Saraswati, "spiritual energy" passes through four different levels of existence — ignorance, sex, love and spiritual experience. In the process of yoga when *kundalini* reaches the fourth centre at the level of the heart, energy is converted from sex to love. When *kundalini* reaches the sixth centre between the eyebrows, the energy is converted from love to spiritual experience. Thus in yoga one's endeavour is to transform sexual energy into love and then to spiritual experience. Pundit Gopi Krishna opined that it is the same energy which is at the two extremes of existence — at the lower level, it is responsible for the erotic experience while at the higher level it gives rise to spiritual experience. The two levels are so close to each other that they appear barely separable from one another.

Elisabeth Haich talks in depth about "sexual energy" and shows the way to convert it into the highest consciousness through yoga.

According to Haich: "Sexuality and the highest consciousness are two different forms in which the one divine creative force, the Logos, is manifested. Sexual energy, the lowest form of the Logos, can in man become the highest form of Logos — divine consciousness. Modern psychology can help us along a part of this path of development but only yoga and meditation can bring us to the goal."

Freud too observed that sexuality can be converted into "spiritually creative power" and he called the process 'sublimation'. Haich points out that the only fuel which is absolutely indispensable for the stimulation of the *chakras* is "sexual energy". The whole process is equally valid for both sexes. The same sexual energy, which has brought man from a spiritual state to a bodily one can bring him back to his divine primal state of wholeness. It is loneliness and not personal relations, which pave the way to God. Yoga is the healthiest and shortest path to

God. One cannot give up sex unless one has known fully what a healthy sex life means.

According to Haich an individual is nothing but one's own sexual energy, which passes through various stages and assumes different forms. "As long as man remains unconscious, he experiences God within himself as sexual desire. When he becomes conscious, he experiences God as his own Self, as his own true being, as I am! God is for man the absolute state of self-awareness." She refers to the union of Logos and the consciousness of the physical being as 'mystical marriage'. Her book shows a picture representing God in Ancient Mexico – at the base is a serpent, symbolising sexual energy; on it stands a man's figure which symbolises the body sustaining emotional, mental and intuitive manifestations; at the very top is the incorporeal, pure spiritual and radiant self-awareness – God. She has noted that the same serpent in India is known as *kundalini* and has described the manifestation of the energy at the seven levels called *chakras*.

It is sexual energy alone which brings us liberation from itself, from sexual energy and from the very sexual desires. It is the cause of inner unrest and it continually goads us to find the inner path. In the words of Haich: "In an unexpected moment, among the animal impulses, in the 'night', in the darkness of unconsciousness, our self-awareness is born. He alone can reach God who has become thoroughly familiar with sexuality and tasted it and all its potentialities to the full, either in this life or in a previous one."

Sexual energy is the bearer of life, and God will remain beyond the reach of a person who is ignorant of sexuality. Full experience of sex can release one from its bondage and then the individual can exercise control over it and use it as a creative power.

Haich observed that a person cannot serve two masters. One can direct the creative powers either to the higher or to the lower centres, not to both at the same time. It means that there is a stage at which the individual stops the use of lower centres and from there only concentrates on higher centres. By this time sexual desire has fallen away from the person like a ripe fruit from a tree. Although the sexual organs are strong and healthy like in any other normal person, the potency goes into a dormant state. Their energy is spiritualised and it is used only in the divine creative way. Truly great persons have never lived licentiously and they have been examples to others on the path of liberation. Pythagoras said that one can either travel the path of spirituality or the path of worldliness, but not both at the same time. The fact is further confirmed with old Hindu teachings. However, it is difficult to find liberated people, as outwardly everyone appears the same. But those who are just below the level of the saintly person can recognise them.

Barbara Harris Whitfield, after journeying herself from sex to spirituality and after interviewing several men and women who had successful experiences, has written the book *Spiritual Awakenings*. According to her, spirituality and sexuality are the two sides of one coin, the coin being our nature. Sexuality is the key to higher realms of transcendent consciousness. People confided in her that their spiritual awakening happened during lovemaking and was preceded by the rush of Divine Energy. Some participants and speakers told her of periods in their journey where they wanted celibacy. The time span she has heard, and practised herself, is a year or two. For some it becomes a permanent choice. Barbara Whitfield observes that the path of intimate relationship may not be for everyone. It may even be inappropriate for some or in some situations. According to her "Divine Energy makes itself known personally. Then two people understand and experience the Sacred Three (God, you and me), becoming one. Union with God is a direct personal experience. Sexuality connects us into a frequency of ecstasy that then connects us back to our Divine Source."

According to psychoanalyst and natural scientist Wilhelm Reich, making love is humankind's attempt to return to the original, unimpeded flow of cosmic energy. Whitfield opines that the blissful moment involves three basic elements — transcendence of time, transcendence of ego and being totally natural. These three things, which give us ecstasy, just happen in sex naturally. Once these three elements have been experienced in sex, one can experience them in meditation too, or vice versa.

Spiritual Sex and Celibacy

According to Whitfield, the science of sex cannot be grasped in a day. Yet, however, persistent efforts can bring results. Her method of spiritual sex is to prolong the act of coitus and remain in the relaxed state while connected genitally, similar to meditation. There should be no thrusting movements except when erection is being lost and then it should be gentle thrusting simply to maintain penetration; full erection is not necessary. The two partners should be at right angles so that the contact is purely genital. There should be no talking and the mind should only be used to sense what is happening. Just feel the flowing warmth, the flowing love and the energy in contact. There should be awareness, without strain, and a feeling of effortless floating. In a short time the valley appears, you have relaxed orgasm and transcendence happens. There is no sex anymore but the meditation of peaceful ecstasy. Von Urban says that the energy cycle becomes apparent and within 28 minutes the bliss sets in and continues for a long time. Barbara Whitfield's talks with others showed that it happens sooner and transcends time. Regular meditation and spiritual sex both last about 20 minutes. There is a renewal of energy and a feeling of being younger, livelier. The key words are 'tension', 'letting go' and 'awareness'.

I have elaborated the fact through a variety of examples that married persons have been more successful in their spiritual quest, in comparison with celibates. Cases are drawn both from the East and the West and from saints to average householders. Many people married more than once in order to find the suitable partner. It may be that people in one way or the other have used "Tantric sex", knowingly or unknowingly.

Osho Rajneesh spent his whole life in perfecting the method of ecstasy, preaching it to others through several centres around the world and he wrote a large number of books on the subject. According to him there is no deeper mystery, no deeper secret, no deeper subject than sex in the world and in life. An average person goes through the routine of coitus throughout his life without knowing what it is. Those souls are rare who understand fully the art of sex, have passed through intricacies of sex and have had rich sex lives in previous births, and are now in a position to attain the stage of real celibacy. Sex has become useless for them and through perfect celibacy they can reveal the truth about sex and divinity.

There are a few valuable observations Osho has made. The first is about the period of coitus. On an average, coitus lasts for about a minute and desire for sex will arise again the next day. If coitus can be prolonged to three minutes, one may not want it again for about a week. A prolongation to seven minutes may extinguish desire for three months and an extension to three hours may free a person for an entire lifetime. Such coitus is *samadhi,* which results in contentment and bliss, which lasts a lifetime.

Perfect coitus leads to real celibacy. In an average person this does not happen and one carries the passion of intercourse to the ripe old age, without satisfaction. Osho's suggestion is to make breathing slow. The faster one breathes, the shorter one lasts in intercourse. Deep breathing through *pranayama* is a way out. Regular practice can bring the stage of sex-*samadhi*, which opens the door to realisation.

The second point is that during the act of intercourse, one should focus attention on the third eye, that is, at a point between the eyebrows. The duration of climax will thus be prolonged, up to even one or two hours or more, and a state of *samadhi* leading to celibacy can be achieved. No one can attain celibacy without the real experience of sex. A successful celibate owes his celibacy to a deep coital union either earlier in the present life or in the previous one. "If during sex one has had an absolute revelation, even once, he is released from sex for the unending journeys of lives."

The third point is to give a sacred status to sex in life. During coitus one is close to God, and as such, one's attitude should be as that of a man going to a temple. If one approaches sex with a pure mind and with a feeling of reverence, one can get a glimpse of the Supreme. Sex is sublimated and bliss is achieved. According to Rajneesh, sex is the re-experience of the original unity. A glimpse of the eternal will convince one that sensual pleasures are meaningless.

The steps to be followed in spiritual coitus can be summarised as follows:

- Develop slow breathing to stay longer.
- Keep your awareness between the eyebrows.
- Have reverence for the Creator.
- Approach sex when you are cheerful, full of love and prayerful.

The temples at Khajuraho, displaying the art of sex and eroticism, near Chhatarpur, Madhya Pradesh, are said to be built by the Chandela Kings of Medieval India. "In the Khajuraho temples is found the juxtaposition of religion and sex. Erotic sculptures on the walls of the Khajuraho temples have religious sanctity and a philosophical background." According to Dey, it symbolises yoga (divine unity) through *bhoga* (worldly pleasures). Tantric scholar Sir John Woodroffe says: "The practitioner is taught not to think that we are one with the divine in liberation only, but here and now, in every act we do, for in truth all Soul is Shakti, it is Shiva, who as Shakti, is acting through the practitioner. When this is realised in every natural function then, each exercise thereof ceases to be a mere animal act and becomes a religious rite, a *yajna* - every function is a part of the Divine Action in Nature."

Brihadarnyaka Upanishada states in a couplet: "In the embrace of his beloved a man forgets the whole world - everything within and without; in the very same way, he who embraces the Self knows neither within nor without."

My observations: The way from sex to Self/ God is straight and short but not so easy. It might take several years or even more than a lifetime, unless the method is understood and applied properly. And, of course, there have been innumerable people who have achieved success in a single lifetime. I would say that sex combined with yogic practices and with reverence to God, and concentration between the eyebrows, which prolongs the duration beyond belief, can bring freedom from sex on the one hand and self-realisation on the other, within a few years in a single lifetime. I have called it regulated sex. This is Tantric sex and has also been professed by Osho Rajneesh as discussed earlier. However, there is another way suggested by Barbara Whitfield through which she achieved success. And, of course, there would be other techniques practised by people over the millenniums.

The stage of "freedom from sex" is clearly known by the practitioner through dreams, visions and direct feelings. For example, one may see in dreams that one's sexual organ is separated from the body like a ripe fruit and a person is putting it at some place in the house. Although one may still desire the company of the opposite sex, there is a great difference. One may desire it for convenience and for the propagation of the teachings and not merely for sex. In fact, if only one of the partners is on the path to God, the other partner begins to complain about the irregularity of sex since he/she still needs it as before.

Self-realisation just happens without warning; one may be in the midst of coitus or doing some routine work. One begins to witness the soul and the manifestation of God in different ways. One may continue to live - eating, drinking, etc., as before, but the inner transformation has taken place. The person may not be recognised as such from the outside because one appears to be the same.

The geniuses in the past used to design methods through which the inner reality could be shown by outer physical symbols for the understanding of the common person. For example, the seven *chakras*, which exist in abstract form on the spine of a human being, have been shown as temples on the Himalayan range, beginning from the temple of Kamakhya Devi in Assam, to the temple of Vaishno Devi in Jammu and ending at the Amarnath temple on top, in Kashmir. Similarly, the inner reality of God-realisation, which is achieved after the annihilation of sex is shown in the temples of

Khajuraho. There one sees erotic scenes on the walls outside and the image of God inside the temple.

There has always been a controversy regarding sex after liberation. It is correct that truly great men have never lived licentiously. According to some, those who have achieved a very high spiritual level and still have sex, although on rare occasions, have not yet become whole; they are on the path of becoming whole. Another view, however, is that if a saintly person once had a physical union with his loved one out of true love, with inner devotion and a healthy physical desire, he should not be considered on any account either a weak, fallen or sinful person. After transformation of the energy one experiences the union of "I" and Logos or *Om* and through "faith and surrender" one lives under the control and direction of the Spirit, having given up self-will. The same Spirit may some time direct one to have physical contact with one's beloved, although the two may be living as celibates normally. After all, even sex is a manifestation of the Spirit.

Summary of the Method of Sex

1. It is the most natural and shortest path to Self/God-realisation.
2. Tantrics tried to transform sex into spirituality, but the preachers of morality did not allow the message to reach the masses.
3. On the faces of the statues of naked people involved in sexual acts, on the walls of the Khajuraho temples in India, one will find the serene and peaceful impression of Buddha and Mahavir.
4. Meditation on these images of intercourse eradicates vulgar sexuality from within and one becomes calm and peaceful.
5. And then when one enters the temple, one finds the peaceful statue of Lord Shiva

engaged in eternal meditation. This is the secret of Tantra. Gaining victory over sexuality leads one to peace and meditation.

6. The process of copulation and orgasm creates egolessness and timelessness, which are the characteristics of *samadhi*.
7. During climax one tastes bliss and divinity.
8. Through proper practice, the *yogi* separates orgasm from ejaculation and then there is no loss of energy and vitality. One experiences mental orgasm constantly and acquires a permanent state of bliss and peace.
9. One has to learn the art of converting sex into meditation.
10. During orgasm the "self" becomes isolated from the lower forces. At this instant, if the man or woman transfers his or her attention from "sensual pleasure" to the "thought of God" or begins to chant a mantra, one day he or she will become aware of "inner awakening" and its associated marks - inner light and sound.

11. Conversion of "sexuality" into "spiritual creative force" is called sublimation, both in man and woman.
12. The same sexual energy which brought one from a spiritual state to the physical body, can take one back to the divine primal state of wholeness through sublimation.
13. For alchemists, "sexual energy" has been the "secret" key to the philosophers' stone.
14. Sublimation is best achieved through the regular practice of yoga, which is the healthiest and shortest path to God.
15. Arousal of *kundalini* is the mark of total sublimation.
16. Sexual energy alone can liberate one from itself and then one becomes a real celibate.
17. When one has mastered the art of sublimation, "self-awareness" is born at an unexpected moment, among animal impulses, in the darkness of unconsciousness.
18. One achieves liberation from the cycle of death and rebirth once for all.

Spiritual Sex - Practical Formula 1

1. Through the regular practice of *yogic* discipline to acquire the power of "holding ejaculation and performing prolonged sex."
2. Chanting of the mantra – *Kling Kling Kling Kamdevaya Namaha* for about an hour every day brings about the power to retain semen for a long time.
3. One should copulate in the state of cheerfulness, love and reverence for the creator.
4. Once penetration is achieved, minimise the act of pulling out and pushing in, as much as possible.
5. Thrusting should be done from time to time only, when one begins to lose erection.
6. Develop slow breathing to prolong the sexual act.
7. Keep your awareness at the mid-point between the eyebrows.
8. Remember God the way you are used to.

9. At the time of ejaculation think that you are sacrificing the semen for a holy purpose.
10. When the right time comes "self-awareness" will be born suddenly and unexpectedly, either in coition or outside it.
11. You will witness inner light and hear inner sound.
12. When this happens the goal of liberation has been achieved.

Tantric Way of Living

Traditionally, tantrics are one of the happiest people with the least number of worries. They have no homes and no fixed shelters, normally living away from human surroundings, having no means of livelihood but whatever would come their way. They are minstrels representing their own spiritual brotherhood. They have friends everywhere and enemies nowhere. They believe in a mysterious binding force that encompasses all living beings and all phenomena, embracing all that is beautiful in life, without getting entangled in their attractions. According to an Indian song, "I take the plunge; I swing in delight; but I keep my head above the water level. No strand of my hair gets wet."

The same thing has been said by the famous sage Shankaracharya: "He who is liberated from the body and is himself perfect, abides in enjoyment like a worldly man full of desires created by past *karma*. But he lives quietly as a spectator, free from desires and changes, like the centre of a wheel." Such people can be seen anywhere and everywhere, anytime and all the time. They preach peace and they mean peace, without troubling anyone for anything. Not caring for anything, they do care for the Soul. They are pictures of unconcern and contentment.

Historical Development of Tantra

A man of peace does not seek peace, rather it is peace that seeks him, and builds a shrine in his soul, which the needy gather for claiming their share. Peace is never sought for selfish satisfaction. An association with a guru normally brings peace into the life of the practitioner, and propels him/her for spiritual perfection. Finding a guru involves faith, which modern people have actually lost. Unfortunately, we became wise at the cost of faith. One, who could provide a packet of peace and pleasure could be a guru. In Vedic times a guru normally maintained a *tapovana* (a peaceful place outside the hustle and bustle of the city), where he would have the practitioners (age 8-20) undergo training for a period of 12 years in order to find the best way of living as a social being. Following an unwritten curriculum, the practitioner would form the basis for life here and beyond. The main purpose of such living was to build up an extremely organised social system, leading to peace within and without. In Vedic times, man's obligations in life were generally chalked out for the entire course from birth to death. The entire cycle of social living was put under expert and strict supervision and guidance. Life was viewed as a planned, orderly span of existence. The man who could provide such training to the practitioners, which could make them use their natural capability, and make them most productive as far as their social demands were concerned was said to be a guru.

A guru is the one who would teach the tenets and practices of *dharma, artha, kama* and *moksha* to the disciples in his ashram. The students at the early age of eight, would be admitted to the *ashram* and would be provided with board and lodging, love and care, and social education which would develop them both intellectually and spiritually. The guru and his family would supervise the practitioners with great care and affection for a period of 12 years.

The four departments of training give a balanced accomplishment to the practitioner. *Dharma* includes the duties to life and beyond, and *artha* prepares one to earn one's livelihood and social prosperity. With this basic training the student is ready to enjoy his natural senses with regard to love, home, aesthetics of art and pleasure, represented by *kama*. Having answered successfully all the demands of body and mind, flesh and spirit, by now the practitioner would be prepared to take a quiet and peaceful departure from the world, represented by *moksha*. Passing from the known to the unknown beyond in a heroic way is represented in many Indian songs. For example: (i) Finish your toilette fast, girl; you are going to meet your beloved.(ii) The locked door has been broken; now delay not beloved; come, O come... The practitioner in India is prepared to cross the barrier successfully and meet the "pilot face to face". He is prepared gradually to say "bon voyage", after living a useful and worthwhile life on earth. This is a courageous and resigned way of meeting death. One happily leaves one's friends and the hall of entertainment like a bridegroom who is going to meet his bride, who has been waiting on the other side. A way to peaceful liberation and happy salvation is shown by *moksha*, which literally means, "the loosening of the bonds."

A person, who could provide such perfect training to the practitioners was called a guru. However, a special instructor would normally be needed at the later stages of training – the one who knows the mysteries and delights of the path of salvation. He is the one who knows both sides well through his personal experiences, and forms a bridge between the immediate worldly life and the eternal life beyond.

To find a guru for these latter stages, the practitioner would leave the homestead behind, severing all the ties, and accepting the life of a forester, called *vanprastha*. Such a living would enable the practitioner to take advantage of the knowledge of hermits who know the secrets of the unknown beyond. One can imagine the great responsibility such a guru would undertake for the sake of others, simply because he loves them as his fellow souls. The life of such a guru is known to be absolutely unimpeachable and sublimated. Such a tradition of Vedic gurus is long gone and forgotten. However, the charm of the Vedic way of living can still be seen in the hangover which mesmerises some diehard optimists, who may still be hoping and trying to bring the old times back into the present.

It was not the ancestral lineage that would automatically pass from one Guru to the next, but the individual's worthiness, which alone would be the deciding factor. In this way the reputation of a guru was protected from being worn out and the indiscreet one would easily be weeded out and thrown away. Some of the respectable and well-known lines of Vedic Gurus are Bhargavs, Bharadwajs, Gautams, Shandilyas and Vashishts. They were known to have unquestionable thoroughness and unblemished expertise. These Vedic gurus were known as teachers in the secular way, and they also acted as priests in religious ceremonies.

Great sacrifices were part of the Vedic life, and such gurus would also conduct these. Buddha also followed one such guru called Gautam, because of which he was later known as Gautam Buddha. However, he discovered that a secular guru did not have the qualities of a hermit and the latter could not satisfy the spiritual yearnings of the former. Accordingly, Buddha left the Vedic discipline and went in search of the truth in his own way and was crowned with success. There were others too with more materialistic views, who were not satisfied with the answers in the Vedic way, and looked for direct knowledge in different ways. The time had changed and another age had begun.

Another example of search, independent of the Vedic method, can be found in Vardhaman Mahavira, who belonged to the princely family of Kshatriyas. He left behind the prevailing norms, rituals and sacrifices and went his own way to find the truth. He was victorious over passion and was called a Jain, and his followers are the present-day Jains. Thus Gautam and Mahavira were the first Protestants of Vedic life, who brought division in the Vedic system, which was well established. From now on, the word guru, which was associated with Vedic rituals and sacrifices, reflected another connotation. The teacher would now be known by different kinds of names, such as acharya and arhat. This brought about the extinction of the Vedic era and the introduction of a "negative philosophy", which could never satisfy the Soul.

The *varna-vyavastha* or caste-system according to which the Brahmins and Kshatriyas were supposed to be superior to others, was disabled. Human classification degenerated to social discrimination. Sacrificial and ritualistic superiority of the Brahmins and the physical superiority of the Kshatriyas was affected. Even in the Vedic period we have heard the stories of clashes between Brahmins and Kshatriyas over the question of superiority. The controversy even broke into pitched battles and the help of learned priests and lawgivers of the time was sought. Vedic society never recovered from this jolt and caste system lost its importance forever.

Sacrifices and the appeasing of the gods was replaced by the cultivation of consciousness and gaining quietude of mind. Mental discipline and ethical order were given importance. Participation with wider forms of life and appreciation of human sufferings began to increase. Unchallenged leadership of the Brahmins in spiritual and religious matters came to an end. The cult of *bhakti* or devotion was developed and God was conceived as a sympathetic member of the human family. *Avatars* or reincarnated Godheads were seriously accepted. Rituals, ceremonies, pilgrimages and holy baths, introduced by Jains and Buddhists, became popular. Auspicious and holy dates in a year were declared. Soothsayers gradually replaced scholars, and priests were consulted for assistance and help in daily life. A new set of gurus began to emerge.

Principles laid down by Jain and Buddhist doctrines entered Hinduism. Terms like *ahimsa* (non-violence), *asteya* (negation of excessive possession and non-sharing), *satya* (truth), *saucha* (cleanliness) and *atmanigrah* (discipline and personal rigours) got introduced into Hinduism. The principles laid down by the sages Kapila and Patanjali got precipitated too and found an honourable place in society. Several social reforms took place such as the abolishing of child marriage and the prohibition of widow marriage and untouchability. The theory of transmigration of souls, reincarnation and the importance of *avatars* gained ground and swept over the whole of Western Asia and the Mediterranean. Brahmanism now became Hinduism, with stress on love and emotion, which could be found in the observance of austerity, fasting, prayer, music and dance.

Bhakti or devotion became the prominent way to God. A personal god or goddess came into being, and the new wave of gurus who could lead people along these lines began. The combined effect of Buddhism and Jainism gave birth to Vaishnavism. Although the famous Buddhist centres of learning, such as Taxila, Nalanda, Ujjain and Avanti were demolished, neo-Brahmanism began to emerge in the South. According to some, this was perhaps because

Egyptian and Iranian Brahmins migrated to India, after political upheavals in that part of the world. Spiritual leadership taken over by doctors and spiritual diviners gradually replaced well-set social orders of the Vedic and Buddho-Jainism periods. Excesses were seen in mysticism and occultism in the form of wine and women being commonly used in rituals.

This was the beginning of the tantric influx on society. It could be because the system of the Brahmins became too scholarly and was filled with austerities and denials. Those who felt a sort of suffocation in the Brahmanical system, found refuge and relief in the more practical tantric system. The message of *bhakti* (devotion) and love through Vaishnavism, coming from the great teachers such as Madhavacharya, Vallabhacharya, Ramanuja and Chaitanya Mahaprabhu began to loosen the system of Brahmanism. The Vedic religion, which prepared the practitioner well for this life and beyond through divine grace, was being taken over by tantric gurus. Gurus in the Vedic period were concerned with the realities and ideals of life here, which would make life in both worlds better. The afterlife was shaped by the deeds in the past, as reward or punishment. They did not talk about the souls outside the body and the related ideas of rebirth and transmigration or ghosts. Pacification of unhappy souls in the afterlife was included in the religious system. Ideals of Buddhism and Jainism were taken over by Vaishnavism, and *bhakti* (devotion) became the chief way of the new Brahmanism. The classless ranks of society began to assemble under the umbrella of *bhakti* with hopes and expectations. Intellectuality, sentimentality, imagination, poetry and music, all combined to give a practical shape to the saying - God is Love or Love is God.

Divine dissension in human or animal form, known as *avatar*, gained importance, and worship of the images of deities became rooted. Although it appeared differently, it was, in fact, the way paved by Buddhism and Jainism. The trinity of Brahma, Vishnu and Mahesh (Shiva) – the creator, sustainer and destroyer – became important. *Bhakti* encouraged the worshipping of personal images and personal redeemers and natural objects, such as rivers, mountains, wells, stones, trees and springs. This was the birth of Hinduism in its present form. There was practically nothing left of the Vedic period – sacrifices, rituals, Brahmins or the sacred gardens called *tapovanas* – no one knew anything about them anymore.

Devotees of all kinds, irrespective of caste and creed, were included in the mainstream of *bhakti* (devotion). The emerging situation was taken care of by the new gurus, who could be called Brahmins in the new form. The devotional practices and the literature coming up now included even the outcastes who were discriminated against by earlier Brahmins. Through devotional practices anyone could enter the mainstream of the Hindu body. Everything appeared logically settled and peaceful. However, the combination of Brahmin priests and rulers of states was becoming a stronghold and the serfs and untouchables continued to suffer, more or less. Nevertheless, devotional practices of *bhakti* created *Swamis* and *Goswamis*, namely the gurus who were masters of their own self, and this was a good boon to society. Under the umbrellas of *Swamis* and *Goswamis*, everyone, without any classification, could grow in the common religious way.

Both Kshatriyas as princes of states, and Brahmin scholars under their protection and sponsorship, were growing in numbers. Vedic laws began to emerge in a new garb of rituals, pilgrimages, holy days and holy nights, art, sculpture, grammar and mathematics. The social order of the country was regenerated by devotion to the Divine and this was nicely reflected in the poetry of the time. The credit for this classlessness of society goes to Buddhism. Nevertheless, Brahmins were the custodians and teachers of religious codes and maintained their importance over others. The logical and metaphysical thinking of the Vedas liberalised the outlook and expanded the mental influence of the practitioners. It is Vedic society which endeavoured to promote human values, enlightenment, peace and illumination, consummating as Self/God-realisation.

The Vedic social system was broken down by the Buddhist way of suppressing the senses and the enjoyments of life. This created an isolated class of people in the world. Submission, tolerance, non-violence, sharing and love became the way to God. The idea of sin from the West got introduced into the system and God was looked at as the sin-washer. Mahayana Buddhism and Svetambara Jainism systematised all these ideas into terms like *urate* (penances), *tirtha* (pilgrimages), *dana* (charity), *snana* (bath) and the feeding of Brahmins. Hinayana Buddhism, supported by spiritual leaders like Shilabhadra, Nagarjuna and Ashvaghosha, influenced the Hindu way of religious life greatly. This was eventually known as the way of Tantra under the new cover of Brahmanism, although it existed much prior to the Vedas. A guru in this system would guide the practitioner into the mysticism of the Unknown, and to the way of getting close to the Unknowable.

References

1. Rawson, Philip 1973. *Tantra*. Thames and Hudson Ltd., London, UK.
2. Rajneesh, Osho n d. *From Sex to Superconsciousness*. The Rebel Publishing House GmbH, Köln, West Germany.
3. Bankroft, Anne 1976. *Twentieth-Century Mystics and Sages*. Penguin Group, London, UK.
4. Saraswati, Swami Satyananda 1984. *Kundalini Tantra*. Bihar School of Yoga, Munger, Bihar, India.
5. Krishna, Gopi 1975. *The Awakening of Kundalini*. Kundalini Research Foundation, New York, USA.
6. Haich, Elisabeth 1982. *Sexual Energy and Yoga*. Aurora Press, New York, NY 10003, USA.
7. Ibid p 49.
8. Ibid pp 54-55.
9. Whitfield, Barbara Harris 1995. *Spiritual Awakening*. Health Communications, Deerfield Beech, Florida, p 135, USA.
10. Kumar, Ravindra 2000. *Kundalini for Beginners*. Llewellyn Publishers, Minnesota, USA.
11. Dey, A.K. n d. *Khajuraho-The Immortal Ancient Sculpture*. Jayana Publishing Co., Delhi, India.
12. Bhattacharya, B. 1989. *Towards a Tantric Goal*. Sterling Publishers Private Limited, New Delhi, India.
13. Chatterji, Mohini M. 1932. *Vivek Chudamani or Crest-Jewel of Wisdom*. The Theosophical Publishing House, Adyar, Madras, India.

Spiritual Series for Beginners

- Bhakti Yoga for Beginners
- Tantra Yoga for Beginners
- Mantras for Beginners
- Karma Yoga for Beginners
- Jnana Yoga for Beginners
- Kundalini for Beginners
- Kriya Yoga for Beginners
- Hatha Yoga for Beginners
- Chakras and Nadis for Beginners